T0368328

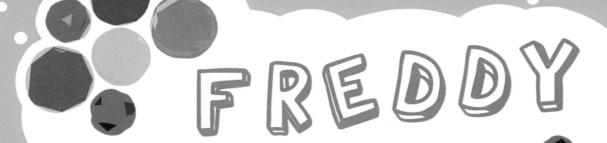

FREDDY

has an ouchy in his tummy

A GLUTEN FREE STORY

Written and
illustrated by
Afarin Faghani

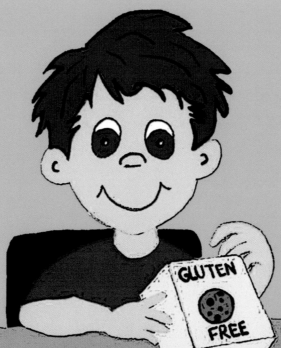

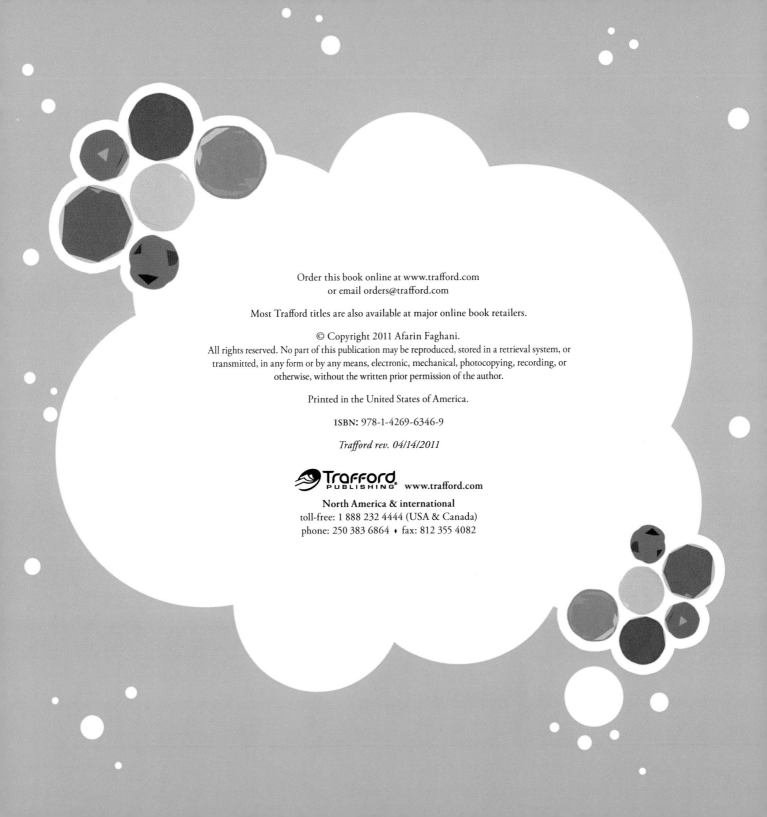

Order this book online at www.trafford.com
or email orders@trafford.com

Most Trafford titles are also available at major online book retailers.

© Copyright 2011 Afarin Faghani.
All rights reserved. No part of this publication may be reproduced, stored in a retrieval system, or
transmitted, in any form or by any means, electronic, mechanical, photocopying, recording, or
otherwise, without the written prior permission of the author.

Printed in the United States of America.

ISBN: 978-1-4269-6346-9

Trafford rev. 04/14/2011

Trafford
PUBLISHING® www.trafford.com

North America & international
toll-free: 1 888 232 4444 (USA & Canada)
phone: 250 383 6864 ♦ fax: 812 355 4082

This book is dedicated to Ellie for her inspiration, my mother for her encouragement; my husband and son for their support.

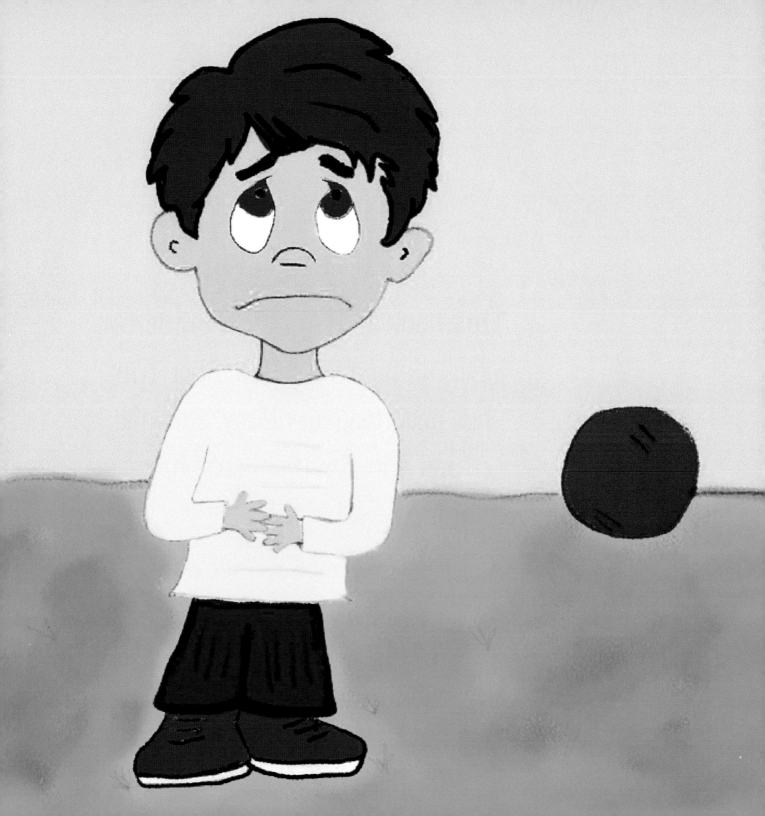

Little Freddy wasn't feeling good.
He had an ouchy in his tummy.
He didn't want to eat or play.

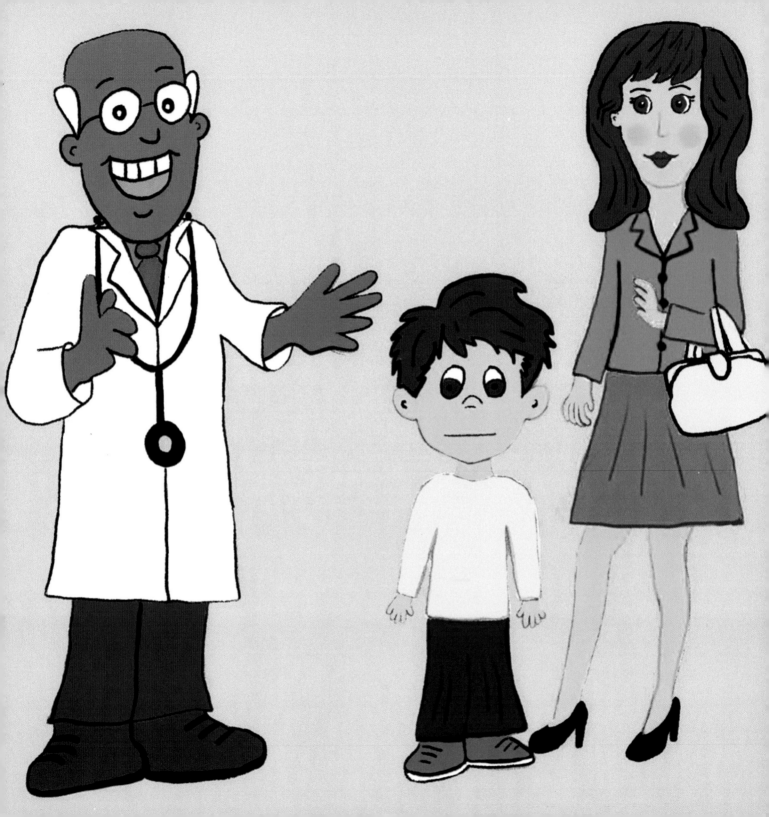

His mommy took him to the doctor. The doctor did some tests and said "Freddy you have Gluten Intolerance". "Glut a what" said Freddy. "Gluten Intolerance" said the doctor again. Freddy wasn't sure what that big word meant.

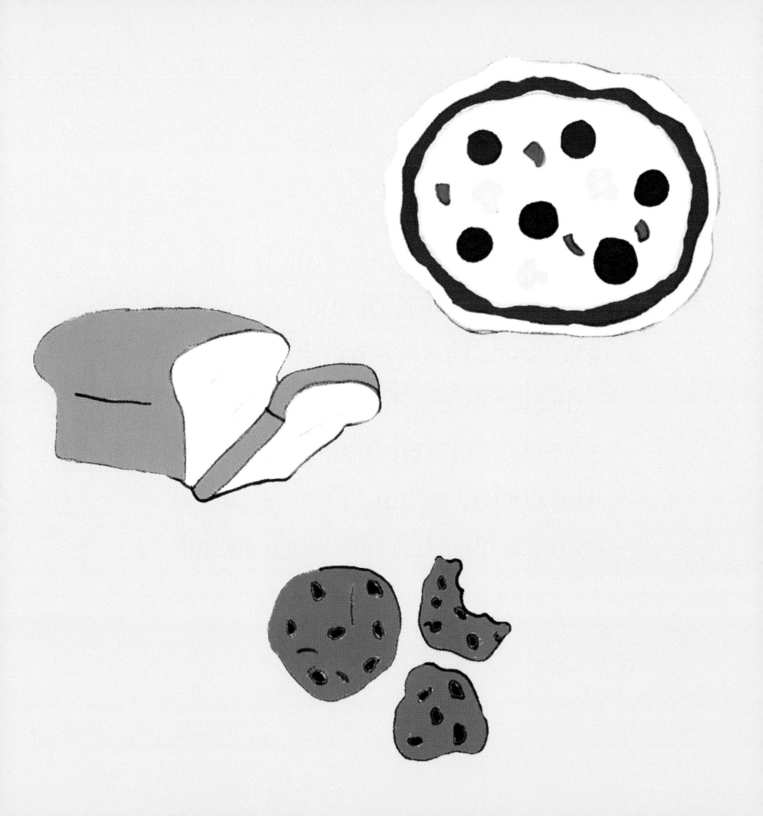

The doctor explained to Freddy that gluten is something in foods made with wheat, rye and barley and his body doesn't like them. That is why he is getting sick. Bread, pizza, pasta, cookies and some other foods have gluten in them so he couldn't eat them.

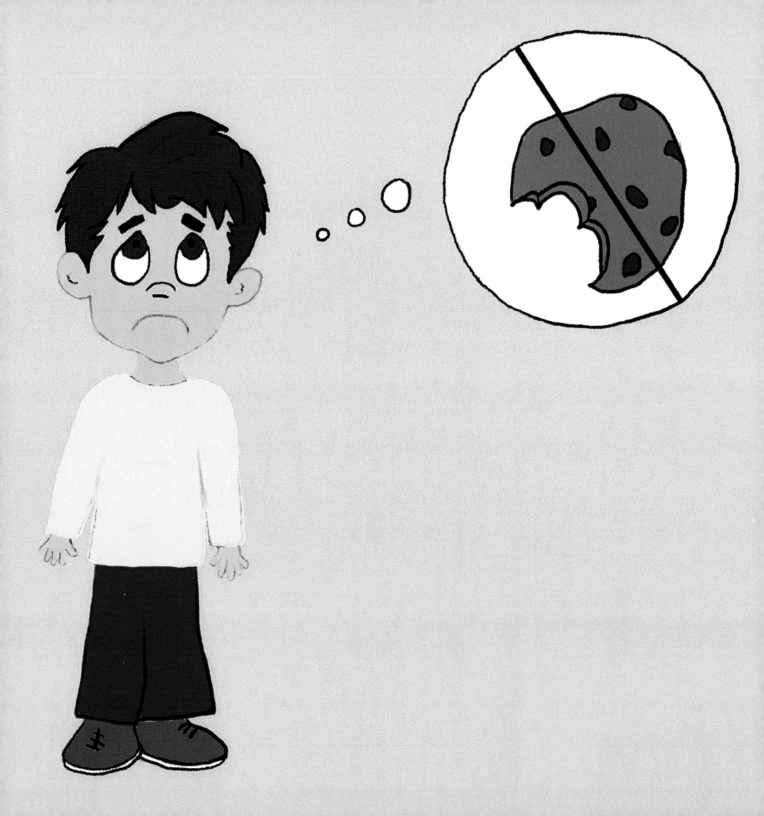

WHAT...NO COOKIES! That made Freddy really sad. How could he NOT eat cookies? They are so delicious!!

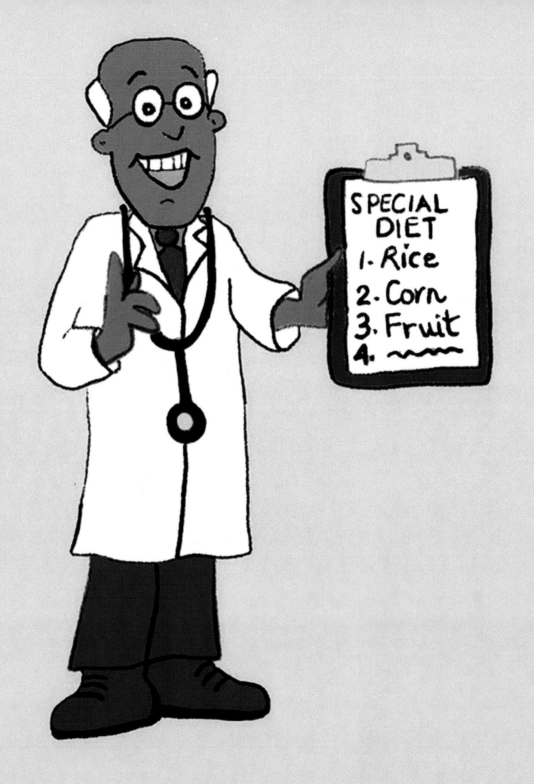

The doctor then said "Freddy, I am going to give you a special diet that I only give to my super brave patients". Freddy was really curious to know what the special diet was. The doctor said "you have to eat foods that do not have any gluten in them, like rice, corn and other vegetables, fruits..." and then he gave Freddy's mommy a list.

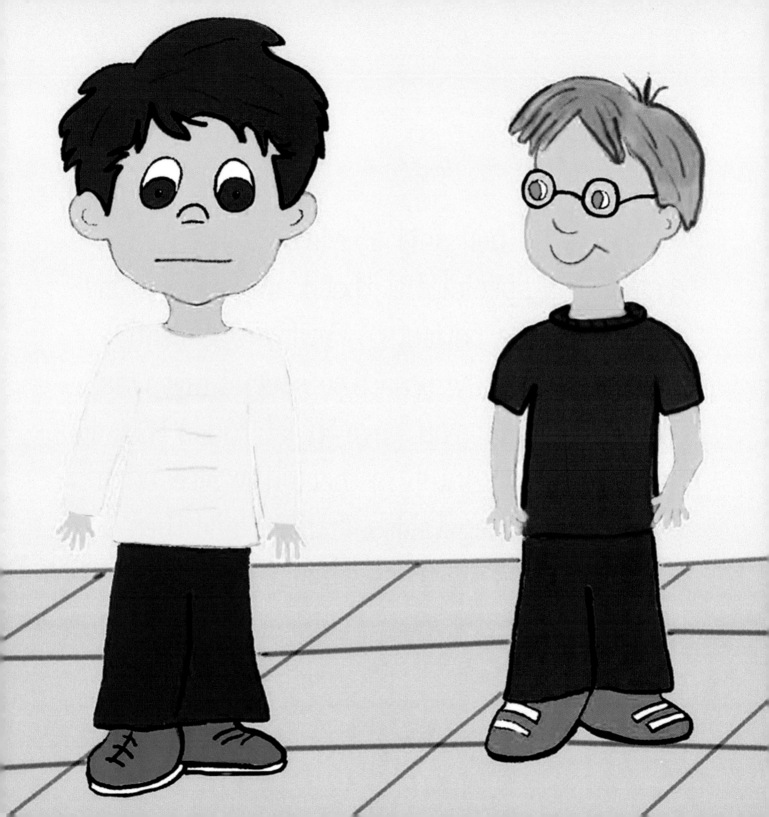

Freddy and his mommy went to the grocery store to buy the things on the list, the gluten free foods.

Freddy wasn't sure what foods he could eat and if they would taste good. At the store, Freddy saw his friend Sam from school.

He was there with his mommy shopping. "Freddy" Sam shouted. "Are you here shopping?" "Yes" Freddy said "I have to buy all new things to eat because I can't eat gluten".

"Me too" said Sam. "I have to eat gluten free foods because I get sick if I don't. Freddy was surprised and happy at the same time.

He was surprised because he didn't know his friend couldn't eat gluten and was happy because he wasn't the only person with gluten intolerance.

A B C D E F G H I J K L M N O P Q R S T U V W X Y Z

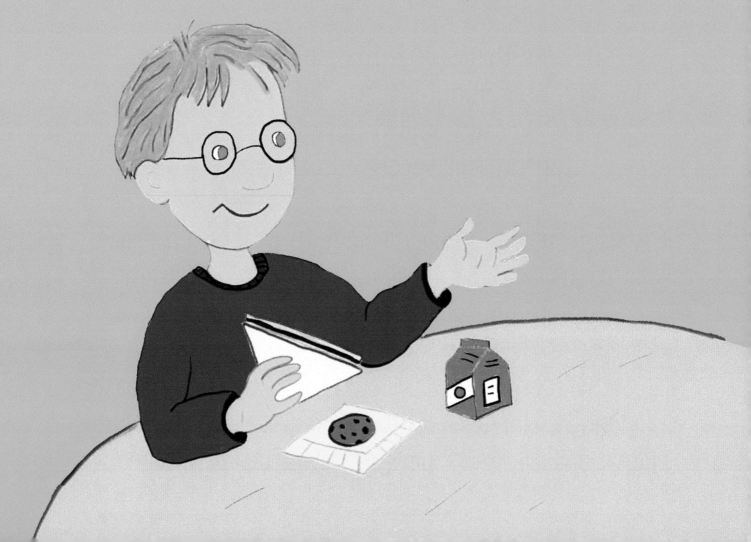

"My doctor said I couldn't eat bread or cookies, but I saw you eat a sandwich and have cookies at lunch" Freddy said. "Yeah, I can't have regular bread or cookies; I have to eat special ones. They taste really good" Sam said. "Here, let me show you where they are" Sam said to Freddy.

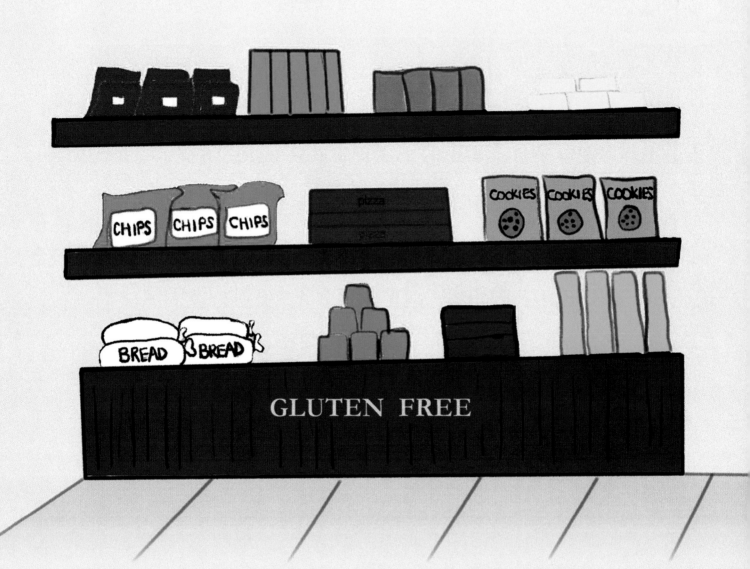

So, Sam and his mommy and Freddy and his mommy all went to the section of the store that was just for people who couldn't eat gluten. Freddy was surprised to see that there was so much food to choose from. Cookies, crackers, chips, cereal, pasta, bread, muffins, pizza and much more. Freddy wasn't feeling sad anymore and he and his mommy picked out all of the special foods he needed for his special diet.

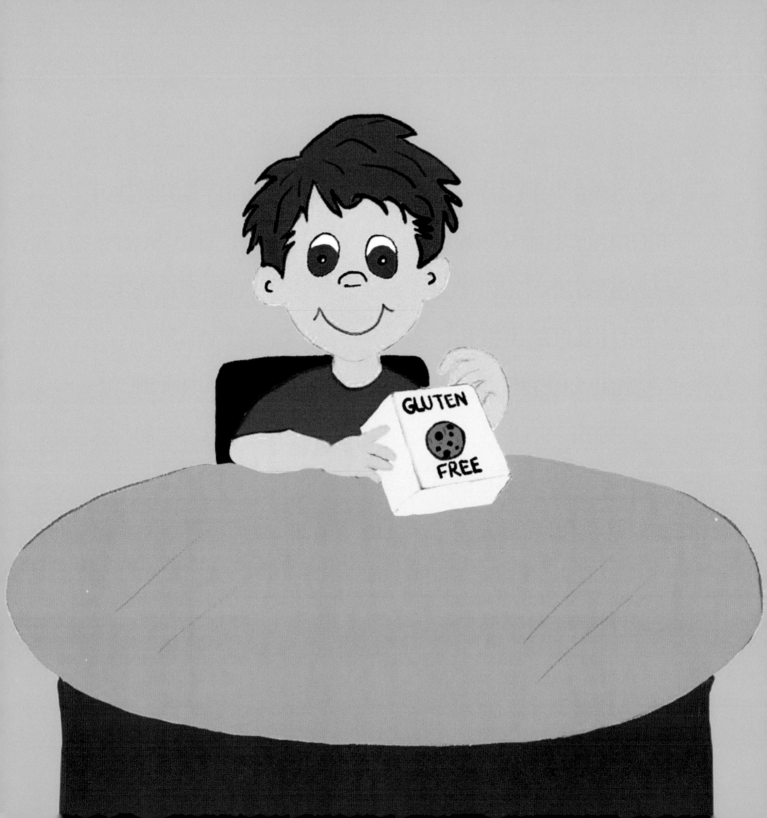

A few weeks later Freddy started
to feel better. He had started to eat
his special gluten free food and
his tummy didn't hurt anymore.
He really liked his gluten free cookies!

Printed in the United States
by Baker & Taylor Publisher Services